Master Cleanse

How To Do A Natural Detox The Right Way And Lose Weight Fast

By Susan T. Williams

This book is designed to provide information on the topic covered. The information herein is offered for informational purposes solely. It is sold with the understanding that neither the author nor the publisher is engaged in rendering legal, accounting or other professional services. If legal or other professional advice is warranted, the services of an appropriate professional should be sought.

While every effort has been made to make the information presented here as complete and accurate as possible, it may contain errors, omissions or information that was accurate as of its publication but subsequently has become outdated by marketplace or industry changes. Neither author nor publisher accepts any liability or responsibility to any person or entity with respect to any loss or damage alleged to have been caused, directly or indirectly, by the information, ideas, opinions or other content in this book.

In no way, is it legal to reproduce, duplicate, or transmit any part of this document in either electronic means or printed form. Recording of this publication is strictly prohibited and any storage of this document is not allowed unless with written permission from the publisher.

The use of any trademark within this book is for clarifying purposes only, and any trademarks referenced in this work are used are without consent, and remain the property of the respective trademark holders, who are not affiliated with the publisher or this book.

FREE EBOOK: 101 SECRETS TO WEIGHT LOSS SUCCESS

available at

www.TheTotalEvolution.Com

Table of Contents

Introduction

We're not always as kind to our bodies as we should be, and even when we make an effort to be healthy the truth is that our bodies are riddled with toxins from an accumulation of bad habits. Sometimes we need to spend some time cleansing our body from all these impurities, and this is where the Master Cleanse diet comes in.

The Master Cleanse Diet is often referred to as the Lemonade Diet, the Cayenne Pepper Diet or the Maple Syrup Diet, however the premise of all these diets are the same. It is a simple 10-day plan through which your body gets a complete detox. During this time, you will lose weight, clean your digestive system and finish feeling happier, healthier and more energetic than you have in years.

The Master Cleanse Diet was originated in 1940 by health practitioner Stanley Burroughs. He developed the cleanse in order to cure a stomach ulcer. He believed that the cleanse worked so well that he published a book in 1976 called The Master Cleanser. The book asserted that the Master Cleanse could help you to not only lose weight but to also cure you from every type of disease. The book had all the right information but it was assembled in a way that was hard to understand.

So in 2004, Peter Glickman – a fan of the diet, put together his own book based on the ideas and principles he had learnt from Burroughs. He named this book 'Lose Weight, Have More Energy and Be Happier in 10 days', and called the diet The Lemonade Diet. Since the release of Glickman's book the diet received much attention and praise and soon saw many people, including many celebrities, giving it a try. Some of these celebrities include Beyoncé and Jared Leto, who both lost a lot of weight at the end of the ten day period.

As with all diets, especially one that is as extreme as this, proper precautions should be taken. In this book, we take a closer look at how you can detox the Master Cleanse way while making sure your body is safe from all side effects. A detox is a fantastic way to lose weight quickly, and if you are doing it the right way, then the results will be great. We'll look at what the cleanse is all about. We'll delve into the health benefits of the detox, and then we'll run through all the frequently asked questions that people have. Most of all, we'll look at how you can incorporate this diet into your life and create the results you want.

CHAPTER 1

The Benefits of Detoxing

Chances are that over the years your body has accumulated its fair share of toxins and impurities. It's not just food that causes this but also the environment that you are in on a daily basis. It's the pollution, the smoke, prescription drugs, chemicals, fertilizers and food additives prevalent in our modern world. Sadly we live in a world where avoiding these issues is almost impossible. We can try to be as healthy as we want, but we still find ourselves becoming contaminated by our environment. When your body is filled with toxins, it is unable to work at its optimal level and all normal functions stop working correctly. You'll find yourself getting tired more easily, putting on weight, getting sick too often, and you'll generally just have a sense of not feeling your best.

Let's take a look at the benefits of a detox:

You'll have more energy. This is certainly one of the greatest benefits from doing a detox and one that might surprise you. You have, more than likely, gotten so used to feeling sluggish that the feeling of being tired is very familiar to you. You might not even see it as a problem because it has become part and parcel of your everyday life. It is only once you finish the detox program that you will understand how unenergetic and lethargic you used to feel. Changing that will give you a renewed sense of energy that you haven't experienced before. You'll have a more natural energy instead of the type of artificial energy boost you used to rely on from caffeine and sugar. The best part of this change is that this type of energy will not result in a sudden crash, and you'll stay energized throughout the day. Having more energy is one of the biggest reasons why people have flocked to this diet because having more energy affects so many other areas in your life. You'll finally feel motivated to do all the things that you want to do, and you'll feel a sense of excitement that you never had before. A person with high energy levels tends to be more successful and is a lot more pleasant to be around then someone who is constantly tired. Friends and family may even note a change in your demeanor and energy levels.

You'll lose weight. Many people go on a detox purely to lose weight fast, and while this is certainly an added bonus, it shouldn't be the only reason to detox, and it should be done carefully. Let me explain: it is only natural that you'll lose weight quickly on a detox because you are suddenly taking in a lot less calories than you're used to. You're also taking your calories in liquid form which flushes your system and causes fast weight loss. However, many people put on the weight that they lost as soon as they stop the detox. That is why you have to be careful with the detox and do it the right way. If you introduce foods slowly back into your diet and allow your body time to adjust then you'll not only lose the weight, but you'll be able to keep it off. We'll run through the detox process later on in the book. Losing weight is certainly a great benefit of the process as it will leave you feeling lighter and more energize. It can sometimes be a great way to kick start a new healthy way of living and give you the boost you need. Another great advantage to losing weight through detox is that you won't feel the heaviness that bad food brings you, and instead you'll feel healthier and more energetic than ever before.

Your skin will shine. When your body is run down from impurities and toxins, your skin remains dull and you'll be more prone to skin disorders like eczema and acne. After a detox cleanse, your skin will feel smoother and healthier and you'll retain a certain glow that you may not have experienced before. This will boost your confidence and help you to look and feel your best. It is important, however, to be advised that the process may not always be pleasant, and you may experience bad skin or itchiness while the detox program is happening. It often takes a while for the impurities to leave the body, and one of the ways in which it does so is through the skin as it is the largest organ in the body. Don't be alarmed if this happens as this is generally a good sign that the detox is working. If you are planning on using this detox to lose weight before a special event than make sure you give yourself enough time for your skin to heal.

You'll get sick less. The problem with a clogged up digestive system is that your immune system is affected, and you are unable to effectively fight any flus or colds that come your way. We've all experienced that feeling of being run down and exhausted only to make matters worse by catching a cold from someone around you. This is because your body is not strong enough to fight back. A healthier and stronger immune system means that your body will be able to absorb nutrients better, and you won't get sick as easily as you did before.

You'll be better at making decisions. A clean and healthy body is directly related to a clean and healthy mind. You'll start thinking more clearly about things, and you'll find that it suddenly becomes a lot easier to make decisions in life. You'll realize that you had been living under a fog for many years.

You'll find it easier to cope with stress. With a cleaner body and a clearer mind you'll find that you are better equipped to deal with any stress that comes your way. Better yet you won't turn to a comfort meal or a bar of chocolate to find release; instead you'll focus on the problem and sort it out. This is because all the nutrients that you will be getting from the cleanse will help keep your adrenal glands calm and nourished and keep you from feeling overwhelmed.

You'll look at your dietary lifestyle in a whole new way. We often get so used to a certain way of living than we don't pay much attention to how healthy or unhealthy it might be. Through years of bad habits most of the things we eat become normal to us, and we don't consider the harm they might cause to our bodies. Once you have finished a detox program, you'll be far more aware of the benefits of a healthy lifestyle, and you'll start to look at yourself and your diet in a whole new way. I know many people who have gone on to become much healthier and happier individuals after a detox purely because they finally knew what it was like to feel this way, and they didn't want that feeling to end. You'll start reviewing your food choices and looking at other ways in which you can create a better lifestyle for yourself. You might eat junk food and suddenly wonder why you even used to like it.

You won't have to reach for the breath mints. It's easy to imagine how bad your breath might be when you consider what is going on inside your body. While you may not realize this yourself you've probably noticed those around you having bad breath. It's not pleasant. When you clear out your digestive system, your entire body starts to function the way it is supposed to and the breath that gets released will be a lot more pure. However, as we discussed with the skin, you may experience bad breath during the detox process. This is simply your body trying to rid itself of all the toxins, and it's a very natural and normal side effect.

Your hair will shine. I always used to say that the way my hair looked was a direct result of the way my body felt. The more run down and lethargic I felt, the more limp and lifeless my hair would be. I would feel the need to wash it more, which would only solve the problem for a little while until it felt unclean again. That is when I realized that the problem had nothing to do with my hair but rather with the health of my body. Once you finish your detox, you will find that your hair starts to regain its shine and will feel soft and light to touch. This is because your hair is finally able to grow freely without being stopped by any impurities that may be holding it back. The better your hair feels the better you will feel.

Lastly, you'll sleep better. It is no wonder that your sleep patterns will be better after a detox, especially considering all the points we have already mentioned. Before the detox you were more than likely suffering from many symptoms which would've stopped you from getting a good night's sleep. Sleep is one of the most important things that a body needs in order to function better throughout the day. Sleep gives your body time to relax and recover from the day and also helps your body to replenish and restore itself. Without sleep your body will not function to the best of its ability. Once your body has gone through a detox process you'll find that you are able to fall asleep with greater ease and you'll experience a better quality of sleep than before. This in turn will have a wonderful effect on the body as it gets ready for the day ahead.

So as you can see the benefits of doing a detox are long and varied, and there is no denying that you will feel better once you've done it. Remember to listen to your body throughout the program and to allow your body time to release itself of all the impurities that have been clogging your system over the years. Now that we know the benefits of a detox, we'll take a closer look at the Master Cleanse and how you can start right now. Your journey awaits.

CHAPTER 2

The Master Cleanse and Lemonade Diet

O kay so now that you've seen the benefits that a detox will have on your body, it's time to show you how to go about the process. The Master Cleanse has some very specific guidelines for you to follow and by following these guidelines for the entire duration of your cleanse, you'll be able to reap all the benefits.

The diet has three phases: The Ease-In to the Master Cleanse, The Lemonade Diet and The Ease-Out of the Master Cleanse.

The Ease-In to the Master Cleanse

As with any new way of eating, it is important to ease into the program rather than trying to immerse yourself in it too quickly and become overwhelmed. In order to do this, you should ease into the diet for the first five days so that it is not a big shock to your system. This will prepare your body for the transformation.

Day 1: Here you can still include food into your diet; however you need to make a conscious effort to regulate what you eat on this day. The focus should be on fresh food as well as raw food. Eliminate all other foods especially any processed food, meat, dairy, alcohol, caffeine or sugar. This is a great introduction to the diet and a good way to prepare your body for what's to come. While day one is optional, it is also highly recommended. Removing processed foods is by far one of the best things to do for your body though it is certainly one of the hardest. Processed food is something the body has not only become used to having, but it is also highly addictive. Processed foods comes in many disguises such as pasta, breads, sauces, fast foods, and all those other treats that have become a natural part of our day. The next step is to eliminate all forms of meat from your diet, which will play a big role in getting rid of that heavy feeling your body has become accustomed to.

Day 2: Day two is all about preparing your body for the full detox ahead. Here you are allowed only fruits and vegetables throughout the day. It is best to look for organic options if possible, though this is not absolutely necessary. Also try to eat your fruit and vegetables raw as opposed to cooking them.

Please note that many people combine day one and two into one day so this is completely up to you.

Day 3: Day three is the day you start a liquid only diet, so it's a great idea to have a blender at hand for this process. Here you can made wonderful juices and smoothies using a variety of fruit and vegetables. You can also liquefy your vegetables to create light soups to enjoy during the day. The most important thing to remember for day three is to make sure that you are only allowing fruit and vegetables into your diet and that you are only consuming them in liquid form.

Day 4: Day four might come as quite a surprise to your system but is an important part of the whole process. This day you are only allowed to drink freshly squeezed orange juice and water. If you feel hungry you can add a tablespoon of maple syrup to the juice, but it is better if you tried to avoid that.

So the first 3 or 4 days will be your ease into the diet, and by now your body will start getting accustomed to this change. Once you have completed these days you will move onto the main section, The Lemonade Diet.

The Lemonade Diet

This is the main phase of the Master Cleanse diet and consists of ten days for you to follow strictly. All the nutrients that you are lacking from food will now be replaced in the form of a lemonade mixture. So for the next ten days, or longer if you wish, these are the guidelines that you need to follow:

No food, fruits or vegetables can be consumed within this period.

Each morning you must start the day off with a salt water flush. This is an important procedure in order for you to eliminate the buildup of toxins in your body. To create this, you must add 1 or 2 teaspoons of non-iodized salt to a full quart of lukewarm water. The amount of salt you use is dependent on what works for your body, but do not use more than 2 teaspoons at a time. This must be taken every single morning on an empty stomach without fail. The salt water flush will create the bowel movement that is needed for the cleansing process. It is important to be aware that your body will react to the liquid quite quickly, give or take half an hour to an hour, so make sure you are in an environment where this won't be a problem. There is no way to make this part of the process sound pretty, and unfortunately it is the only way your body is going to release itself of all waste. You might have to rush to the bathroom a few times until you feel clear of everything. As I said, it's certainly not very pleasant, but you'll feel so much better because of it.

You must drink 6 or more glasses of the Master Cleanse Organic Lemonade mixture. You can do this throughout the day. You can make this by blending 2 tablespoons of fresh lemon juice, 2 tablespoons of rich Grade B Maple Syrup, 1/10 of a teaspoon of cayenne pepper and 1 – 2 cups of fresh water. Make sure that you do not store your lemons in the fridge as this will kill the enzymes that your body needs. Also, don't think you can skip the lemons and use lemon juice instead. It is imperative that you use fresh lemons for this. For the water, make sure you are using fresh water and always look for the best quality you can find. Also, make sure that you drink your lemonade mixture fresh, so don't make a lot and store in the fridge for the day. It's better to drink it as soon as you make it. Lastly, make sure to spread your 6 glasses throughout the day, and don't try to drink it all at once. If you are more worried about losing weight than about the detox process, then decrease the maple syrup to one tablespoon instead of two.

End each day of the Lemonade Diet with a herbal laxative tea. This will help with the elimination process and help speed up the detox. It is up to you what type of laxative tea you want as there are quite a few available on the market.

Before we move on to the final stage of the Master Cleanse, let's take a look at how your body might feel during the ten days:

Day 1 – 3: These are the hardest of all the days as your body is going through a complete elimination process that it has not experienced before. You will feel tired, upset and you'll be running to the bathroom a lot. This is normal. Remember that your body is trying to release itself from years of bad toxins.

Day 4 – 5: Finally, you'll start to see a light at the end of the tunnel and you'll start to emerge from the fog that you've been living in. You should start to feel a lot more stable than you did in the first few days and you'll start experiencing more energy that what you are used to.

Day 6 – 7: By now you've probably had enough. You've gone through highs and lows and you are thinking about food a lot more than you should be. It's important to keep yourself busy through these two days.

Day 8 – 10: Ah, you're feeling better again as you reach the end of the road. You're happier and you are starting to feel the benefits of the diet. Your skin has cleared, your hair feels soft, your body feels light and you feel energetic. By day ten, you're ready to start the ease-out process and you're looking forward to starting a healthier lifestyle.

The Ease-Out of the Master Cleanse

Once you are done with the ten days of the Lemonade Diet, you will start to ease out of the Master Cleanse process. This is important, as it will help your body to maintain the weight that it has lost and will help you to easily adjust back to a normal way of eating.

You do not want to go straight from here into normal eating as it will be a shock to your body, and the reaction might not be pleasant. Also if you skip the ease out process, you will more than likely put back on all the weight you have lost, and the whole experience would have been for nothing. The whole point of this carefully designed detox is that you are smart about the decisions you make in order to sustain a long-lasting effect.

Day 1: Drink only orange juice. You will remember doing this as you were easing into the process, and the same principles will apply. You will find it easier to maintain this second time around because you won't be going from foods to orange juice so quickly. After ten days on the Lemonade Diet, you should find this day a lot easier to manage, and you'll be used to the acidity a lot more. Remember to opt for freshly squeezed orange juice and to drink it slowly throughout the day. The process of drinking orange juice straight after the ten-day detox is important as it gets your body ready to digest food again. Remember to also drink a few glasses of water on this day, too.

Day 2: You'll carry on drinking freshly squeezed orange juice and water throughout the day, however, this time you'll add vegetable soup to the diet as well. The vegetables must be freshly prepared (so nothing from a can), and you can enjoy this twice in the day, consuming mostly the broth and a few of the vegetables. While you are allowed a few vegetables on this day, you should try not to overdo it.

Day 3: Drink a glass or two of freshly squeezed orange juice in the morning. Later on you can enjoy some more of the vegetable soup that you made the day before, and later on that evening you can have any vegetables or fruits. Please note that while you are now off the detox diet, it is still important to stick to the schedule and not jump into normal food too quickly. So today is all about slowly introducing more solids into your diet throughout the day.

Day 4: Now you are back to a normal day of eating. However, normal now does not mean what it did before. Take it slow and keep in mind that your body needs food that with nourish and sustain it.

The most important thing to consider throughout the entire process is learning how to ease your body into a new and healthy lifestyle. This will help you to maintain your results, and it will be much gentler on your body.

Using the Master Cleanse as a means to lose weight

It is vital that you are fully aware that this is not a dietary lifestyle. It is not something that you can do for the rest of your life. This is a short detox plan to help rid your body of toxins, flush out your system and rid yourself of unnecessary fat. It is step *towards* a healthy lifestyle and a kick start in the right direction. A lot of the weight that you lose throughout the process will be a buildup of fecal matter from years and years of bad eating or unhealthy habits. In addition, you will also lose a lot of water that your body has been retaining. The intention of the Master Cleanse is not only to lose weight but rather to clean your body from all the impurities and to set your mind right through the detoxification process. Through a clean mind and a clear head, you will then focus on creating a healthy lifestyle for yourself, and you'll continue to lose weight in a slower but more natural way. See the Master Cleanse as a step towards your ultimate goal but not the goal itself. There is a lot you will learn throughout this process, and it is important to take those lessons with you as you continue with your normal day-to-day life. Start creating better habits for yourself, and do the Master Cleanse a few times a year for best results. You can time it so that you do the Master Cleanse at the beginning of each season.

CHAPTER 3

The Three Main Ingredients

The three main ingredients of the Master Cleanse diet are lemons, cayenne pepper and maple syrup. They were each chosen with a specific purpose to help with the detox process. Let's take a closer look at what they are all about:

Lemons

Lemons are one of the most important naturally produced foods that we should be including into our daily diet. While you will consume lemons daily throughout the ten-day process, it is important that you continue to enjoy them even when your detox is done. They are very versatile and contain so many amazing healing properties for the body. So why are lemons so good for you?

They are packed with vitamin C, which means they will improve your immune system and help you to fight off viruses including colds and the flu.

They give a natural boost of energy and, unlike other stimulants, they do not cause a crash later on.

They have a diuretic effect on the body and will help to flush out all the impurities from your system.

They are used in the treatment of kidney stones. By introducing lemons into your system early enough, they may even save you from having to get kidney stones medically removed.

Just a few drops daily will help with indigestion and constipation.

Lemons are great for your skin and can even be applied directly to sunburn, blackheads and eczema.

Cayenne Pepper

Cayenne pepper is a natural spice that not only adds great flavor to meals but also has many incredible properties for the body. Here are some of the health benefits it has:

Cayenne pepper works wonders to ease an upset stomach.

It will help with a sore throat or a persistent cough.

It lessens the pain caused by a migraine headache.

It works wonders for the digestive system, as it increases the flow of enzyme production and helps the body to better metabolize food and to better release unwanted toxins.

It causes people to sweat, which will help greatly in the detoxification process, allowing the body to rid itself of impurities with ease.

It is great for people who are trying to lose weight. Including cayenne pepper to your breakfast each morning causes you to stay fuller for longer which means you'll take in fewer calories throughout the day. It also increases the metabolism so that you'll burn off those calories even quicker.

Maple Syrup

The type of syrup that is used in the Master Cleanse diet is Grade B Maple Syrup. It has a very high vitamin content and will help to replenish the body of any nutrients that it might lose during the elimination process. Grade A Maple Syrup goes through quite a strong refinement process, which strips it bare of all its naturally good components. This is why only Grade B maple syrup is allowed in this diet.

Maple Syrup is created by boiling the sap of the sugar maple tree in very big shallow pans over a hot fire. It has all natural minerals and vitamins including B2, B5, B6, Biotin, Folic, Calcium, Magnesium, Iron, Phosphorus, to name a few. It has been dubbed a 'superfood' and researchers are now urging people to include it in their diet. Some of its health benefits include:

It has many antioxidant and anti-inflammatory properties which help with fighting many illnesses, including cancer. It also plays a big role in helping to prevent prostate cancer in men.

It helps build up the immune system as it has a strong component of zinc and magnesium.

54 beneficial compounds have now been identified by researchers in the field.

CHAPTER 4

Tips and Tricks

There's no denying that embarking on a detox is not an easy process, and you'll certainly encounter many highs and lows throughout the process. It's always great to have support, which is why I've put together this list of tips and tricks to help you get through it:

Decide on the date that you want to start the detox, mark it on your calendar and make sure that you have put it somewhere where you can easily see it. You want to be reminded that you have made this decision, and you can use the upcoming days to prepare for the start of your cleanse. Try to plan your detox around a time that isn't too busy as you don't want to be going to a wedding or a birthday party or something similar during this time. Be smart about your decision to start, and make sure it is best for you.

Prepare all your ingredients before you begin. Make sure you have all that you need to ease you into the diet as well as for the ten-day process itself. It is important that you feel both mentally and physically prepared for the challenge. The easier you make it for yourself, the easier it will be to complete the cleanse and see it through to the end. Establishing a set routine will help you, and many people have found that writing out the diet in a step-by-step guide and sticking it to your refrigerator or somewhere else in the kitchen has helped them to be constantly aware of what they need to do. Tick off each day as you do it, so that you know where you are. It will give you a sense of relief at the end of the day to see yourself ticking off another day and knowing that you are slowing approaching the end.

Start off correctly. Make sure you know exactly what you need to do as soon as you get out of bed. Wondering what you have to do for the day might leave you confused and annoyed. Instead know your structure. Most of the time this means starting off the day with either water, orange juice or the lemonade mix, depending on what day you are on. Starting the day off in the right way and with the right frame of mind will set you up nicely for the rest of your day. Start off strong, and end strong. This is a trick that athletes always use. The night before a race they will prepare everything and set it out next to their bad. That way as soon as they get up they can simply put on all their gear and have all their accessories at hand. This takes away any stress or confusion in the morning and guarantees that you will start of the day in a more positive mindset.

Do your research. After reading this book, go ahead and spend some time online getting as much information as possible. It's always great to see what others have gone through and experienced in order to answer any questions you might have. Knowing that others have gone through the same thing is always a great motivator. There are also hundreds of forums online where you can join a conversation and ask others questions.

Visit your doctor. Don't be afraid to chat to your doctor before starting the process. Sometimes speaking to someone that knows your medical history can be extremely beneficial. If you have any questions it's best to get them answered so that you can feel safe and happy when you decide to start the detox.

Have a set schedule. A lot of people say that this is one of the biggest things that helped them throughout the ten days. They created a schedule which detailed exactly when they need to have a drink. This way they were able to curb their hunger and keep their temptations at bay.

It's best not to exercise throughout the detox. If you are already a very active person, and you don't want to give up your exercise, then make sure you keep the exercises light and easy. Don't push yourself too hard throughout this period. Remember that your energy levels will be low to start, and you will not be getting any extra nutrition from food. If at all possible, try not to resume exercise until the easing out period. Be gentle to your body in this time, as you don't want to put yourself under any unnecessary stress.

Stick it out, and be strong. The first three days are the hardest, so if you can get through those first days, then you will definitely be able to do the rest. Start off knowing that it is going to be hard, but be strong in your will to keep going. It is always better to be prepared and to be honest with yourself at all times. Knowing how hard it is going to be but understanding that it is not forever, is a great way to keep yourself strong throughout the process. You'll be surprised at just how much you can do and how strong your will and your mind can be, if that's what you truly desire.

Plan activities throughout the day. It's important that you try to keep your mind as occupied as possible so that you are not constantly thinking about the diet or how hungry you are. Your mind is a powerful tool if you use it correctly. Have you ever needed the toilet so much that it was the only thing on your mind? Then suddenly something happened to distract you and an hour went past, and you realize you had completely forgotten that you needed the toilet. This has happened to me so many times, and I'm always so surprised that I was able to forget a feeling that was previously so powerful. The power of distraction is key to making you get through this diet. So, plan lots of activities and keep yourself busy. The more you think about food, the hungrier you will be. So fool your mind into thinking about something else, and you'll be able to get through the day with ease.

If you're not going to be at home, then make sure you pack a cooler filled with whatever you will need for the day. While it is always best to drink your lemonade mix as you make it, this might not always be possible each and every day. If you are not going to be sitting at home all day or in an office environment that lends itself to flexibility, then pack your bag with what you need, even if this means preparing your juices before you leave. When you make the juice, be sure to take the cayenne pepper separately and add that to the serving when you drink it and not before. The maple syrup acts as a preservative which will keep your juice staying fresh for longer. Always try to stick to the diet as strictly as possible, but if you can't, then find a way to work around it, and don't stress yourself out unnecessarily.

Ask your friends and family to support you. One of the biggest reasons that people fail on this diet is their inability to remain strong while having to cook for their family or while going out with friends. It is important to let those around you know what you are doing and to ask them for their support. If anyone can help you through the cooking process that would be great, but if not then make sure that they know what you are doing and why you are doing it. Remind yourself that the cleanse is not for long and that the entire process will be over soon. It's good to let friends and family know not just what you are doing but why you are doing it. If they know just how much it means to you, then they will be more willing to help you through this process.

See if anyone wants to join you on the diet. While it's great to have support from those around you, it is even better to do the diet with someone else. Having someone to do this with will make the process so much easier as you can lean on each other for help and support. Make sure you start the process together and do the same steps each day so that you will not only start together but also end together. You'll be tempted to cheat, so having someone doing it with you will be a great way to get through those feelings. It's also an added bonus to have someone to celebrate with at the end, especially someone who has experienced all the same emotions that you have throughout the process.

Keep a record of your progress. This is a very interesting experiment to do throughout the detox. By tracking everything you eat or drink and when you do it you will be able to keep a good record of the entire process, which means you won't forget how many drinks you have had, etc. Also, by writing down not only what you had but also how it made you feel you'll get a better understanding of your body. You'll start to understand what your body needs and what it doesn't need. Too often we go through life without really listening to our body, and we remain blind to what it is telling us. By becoming more aware of your body you will be able to use these skills throughout your life in order to give it what it needs.

Stay hydrated. You're going to have moments when you feel weak, tired and shaky. This is only natural as it is your body's way of trying to adjust to not having processed food. You always feel worse before you feel better, so it's important to be aware of this and keep it in mind as you do the cleanse. Throughout the process, make sure you are properly hydrated. This means drinking a lot more water than you normally would. Remember that your body is going to flush out a lot of waste, and you will be losing a lot of water during this time, too. So make sure you are giving yourself extra water to account for any liquid that you may lose. Keep drinking the drinks that you are supposed to drink on that particular day, and remember that they are an important part of the process. You may not enjoy the taste or the sensation, but remember again, this is just a ten-day detox and not something you will be doing forever.

Weigh yourself. You are going to be losing weight throughout the Master Cleanse, and by weighing yourself daily you will found the motivation to carry on and keep it up. It's not uncommon to find yourself becoming despondent through the process, especially if your body has become used to processed food. So weighing yourself might just give you that pick me up that you need to see you through. At the same time, don't become despondent if you don't see weight loss immediately. While most people lose weight quite quickly, others take a bit longer to see results. Everyone is different. But continue to weigh yourself regardless as you WILL eventually see the progress you are looking for.

Create a reward system. While feeling good and losing weight is certainly a reward in and of itself, it can sometimes be worthwhile to create a separate reward for yourself in order to keep you motivated throughout the whole process. Perhaps you'll treat yourself to a quick weekend trip, to a new outfit or to a day at the spa. Do whatever it is that suits you and your lifestyle, and keep yourself motivated. I heard a great story about someone who put aside ten dollars at the end of each day in an envelope marked 'me time', and by the end of her detox she enjoyed a full day aimed at completely spoiling herself. She knew she worked hard, and she knew she deserved it. Doing something like this is a great motivator to see you through.

Enjoy your sleep. A detox is definitely going to help you to feel more energized than you ever have before, but this is only going to come into effect once you have finished the program or at least are close to the end. In the beginning, you are going to feel tired and lethargic. This is natural as your body is trying to figure out what to do without all the food that it is used to getting. Sleep is your friend in this process. Not only will you want to sleep more, but the sleep will help to ward off the hunger pangs. Give your body the rest it needs, and use your sleeping time to your advantage.

Remember why you are doing the cleanse. It can often become easy to forget the reason behind starting the detox in the first place. Heard of the common phrase 'hangry'? It is a clever combination of words meaning that you are angry because you are so hungry. This is something everyone has been through at one stage of the cleanse and something you will feel a lot throughout the detox. This feeling of anger can sometimes get in the way of the process, and you might feel the need to pull out and quit. Don't. Take a deep breath and ask yourself why you are letting food get in the way of your emotions. You need to start seeing food in a different way and realize that you should have control over it and not the other way around. Whenever you find yourself getting hangry just take a deep breath and remember the reason you started this process. Count how many days you have left and understand that not only is this not forever, but by the end you'll be a healthier and happier version of yourself. You will never get where you want in life without patience, perseverance and hard work. Constantly motivate yourself, and find your inner strength. You won't be sorry. If fact, you'll be glad you did.

Lastly, a friend of mine recently did the Master Cleanse, and I finally managed to catch up with her a few days after she finished. I knew she was doing the detox, but even though I tried to stay in contact, I saw very little of her throughout that time. I assumed she was busy and didn't think much of it. I was excited to finally see her. She looked great, and I asked her what tips she could provide.

She said: *'I'm going to be honest with you. I'd like to pretend that the whole thing was a breeze and that I didn't think about food at all throughout the process. But I'd be lying. It wasn't easy. If you are wondering why you haven't seen me for the past two weeks it's simply because I wasn't in the mood to see anyone, and I certainly didn't want to be reminded about food. I was angry in the beginning and kept wondering why I was doing this to myself. I wanted to quit. But I had taped a note to myself which I saw every day when I looked in the mirror. It said 'You're not just doing this for yourself. You're doing this for your kids.' That kept me going. I wanted to lose weight and have more energy so that I could feel better about myself. But mostly I wanted to be the best mom that I could be for my kids. I was quite frankly tired of always being tired. The diet wasn't easy, but I was motivated and I got through it. It's amazing what you can do when you really put your mind to something. It helped having a goal to work towards. Also, I knew that I had told quite a few people that I was doing this, and I knew they would all be asking me how it went and holding me accountable. I didn't want to embarrass myself and tell them I had quit. So I kept on going. I'm feeling much better than I have in years, and I'm quite determined to carry on towards this healthy lifestyle.'* I then asked her if she missed pizza and cake (which I knew were her two favorite things) and she laughed, *'Of course I do. But I keep reminding myself that my life and my health are far more important and those feelings kind of take over. Yeah I still want cake, but I want to look and feel good a whole lot more'*.

CHAPTER 5

Frequently Asked Questions

As with everything in life, the more you do something, the better you'll get at it. It is just the same with the Master Cleanse diet. You might battle with a few things the first time around, but when you do it again a second or third time you'll learn from some of the mistakes you made the first time. Luckily, I'm here to help you. Below are some of the traps you might fall into on your first try. I've rounded up some of the most commonly asked questions that people who are trying out the diet for the first time tend to ask.

How do I know if my body is craving something or whether I'm just bored?

Knowing when you're truly craving something or not is not as easy as it might sound. This may seem silly at first and you might be thinking 'well if I'm craving something then I obviously want it'. The truth is actually quite different, and craving doesn't always mean that you're hungry. There are many other reasons why you might be craving something. Sometimes you're craving a particular type of food because your body is lacking in a certain nutrient. Or sometimes you are craving food in order to fill an emotional or psychological gap. The problem with this is that food will only help you while you are eating it, and after that you'll continue to feel the same way. That is why the cleanse is so important, because it will help you to better recognize the signals that your body is giving you and will force you to face and overcome any other food issues you might have.

Can I buy any type of maple syrup?

Although there are a few disagreements on this topic, the original diet states that only Grade B maple syrup should be included. This is because you are looking for a syrup that is pure and unrefined in order to get the best results. It is in your best interest to look for the purest and most natural maple syrup that you can find so that you can get the most nutrients into your diet as possible. Plus, it tastes great, which is an added bonus.

Can I stay on this diet for longer than the recommended 10 days?

This is completely up to you, however research has shown that ten days is usually sufficient. Remember that you will be easing into the diet for a few days as well as easing out of it, so the entire process takes just over two weeks. Do not attempt to do more than ten days if this is your first time trying out the cleanse. Personally, I do not think you should try to stay on this detox for too long. Instead, do it for the recommended number of days, and do it three or four times throughout the year, for example, at the start of each new season. This will give you optimal results.

Is this a diet or a detox?

Ultimately this is a detox. It is a way for your body to cleanse itself from any residual impurities that it has stored up over the years. However, because you will walk away with a greater sense of your body and your health this can, in a way, be considered a diet of sorts. Continuing to include lemons, cayenne pepper and maple syrup in your diet after the cleanse is over is a fantastic way to keep healthy and a great thing to do on a day-to-day basis.

Can I take supplements throughout the detox?

The detox was designed so that throughout the ten days you get all the nutrients you need. Supplements should be avoided so that the natural process of the cleanse is not interfered with. However, every person is different, and it is important to do what feels right with your body. If you are unsure, then it is perhaps better to speak to your doctor before making a decision.

How much weight will I lose?

Every person is different, and it is impossible to accurately determine how much weight you will lose. On average you should lose around 2 – 3 pounds in the first two days and then 1 pound per day until you finish. Of course, this is largely determined by how much weight you need to lose in the first place.

How many bowel movements are considered normal?

You should experience 2 – 3 bowel movements a day, although some people experience a lot more at the beginning until their body starts to adjust.

How hungry am I going to be?

To be honest, the detox was created so that you would not get hungry because you are going to get all the nutrients and calories that your body needs. If you do feel hungry, it is more than likely due to what you are used to eating and is your body's way of feeling confused without the food. Or, if you are an emotional eater, you might feel as if you are hungry simply because you are used to feeding your emotions with food. It's important to use this time to really get to understand your body and grasp why it is sending you these signals.

Do I have to use cayenne pepper? I really don't like it.

Adding loose cayenne pepper to your lemon water is the preferred method throughout this detox. However, if you need an alternative, you can have cayenne capsules instead. In that case, you would be looking at taking between 3-4 100mg capsules a day.

Can I have a cheat day?

No, you cannot have a cheat day on this diet, especially since it is only ten days for the detox period. There are no shortcuts with this diet, and if you want to see the best results, then you need to follow it exactly. When you start this cleanse you have to understand that it is not going to be easy, and you have to make the decision from the start that you will stick to it no matter what. Don't let other foods stop you from achieving your goals, and never lose sight of your dream. Not only will you gain the full benefits by sticking it out, but you'll enjoy a greater sense of achievement for not giving up.

Can I skip the easing in or easing out process and just do the ten days?

No. This cleanse has been well formulated and researched to make it easier and healthier on your body by having an adjustment period. Your body needs the time to ease into it, and your body also needs the time to ease out of it. Again, try not to think of taking shortcuts. If you do the entire thing properly, you will feel great, and you will have gained so much more from the experience.

Can I continue with my normal life throughout the cleanse?

Yes, absolutely. You can continue to do all the things you would normally do on a regular day-to-day basis. The only time that you will want to stay close to home is for the first few days on the diet. Here you'll be feeling weak and tired, and you might need to rush to the bathroom at short notice. After the initial few days, you'll be back to normal and can resume all activities.

Are there any side effects?

Yes, but they vary from person to person, and most of the side effects only happen in the first few days. Some of these can include weakness, lethargy, hunger pangs, headaches, anxiety and diarrhea. You may also find you are a bit more emotional in the first few days as your body tries to make sense of what is happening. This is normal, and these symptoms should subside quite quickly.

Can I do this even if I am diabetic?

If you are concerned about a medical condition, it is best to first check with your doctor before embarking on the cleanse. You will be able to do the detox if you are diabetic, but it is best to check with someone who knows your medical history to see if this is the right route for you or if any adjustments can be made to suit your body.

Can I do this if I am pregnant or about to have surgery?

No, this detox cannot be done if you are pregnant, and the same goes for anyone that is going in or coming out of a surgery.

Can I still smoke?

No. In order to get the full benefits of the cleanse, you need to eliminate any harmful substances from your body. You're on this detox because you want to lose weight and because you want to create a healthier and happier body and mind. If you are a smoker, then perhaps now is the time to take a closer look at why you are smoking and use this as an opportunity to quit. Use these ten days as a complete holistic experience, and at the end ask yourself if you really want to continue smoking again.

I don't like the taste, can I use anything other than maple syrup?

You should try to stick to the maple syrup as much as possible, however if you really cannot stomach it then you can use molasses instead. Or if you can get your hands on freshly squeezed sugar cane juice, then you can use that. However, try to stick it out with the maple syrup as it will work the best.

Is the diet safe?

The diet consists of only pure and natural ingredients. It has absolutely no preservatives and no artificial colors or flavors. It is a safe way to flush out toxins and will also give you enough calories to see you through the week. Unlike other cleanses, this detox also includes an ease in and ease out period to make sure your body adjusts well to the process.

Conclusion

Thank you again for downloading this book!

A detox is often a very necessary thing to go through in order to jumpstart your body into a healthier and happier way of living. You can do this a few times throughout the year to make sure that you are constantly ridding your body of all excess waste. Let's be honest, life can be so busy that we often forget just how important it is to cultivate a healthy body and mind. A detox is a great reminder of how necessary it is to have a fully functioning body in order to live a better life. The Master Cleanse diet will be a great start for you as it has clear and defined instructions. By following these guidelines, you will end the process feeling so much better than you ever have before. Not only will you restore your body with fresh nutrients, but you'll also lose weight and look amazing in the process. Quite frankly, you owe it to yourself to take on this challenge and to do it well!

This is a very popular diet because it is seen as a step towards a better life rather than just a fad diet that will come and go. Most people who have done it once say that they would definitely do it again. One of the best parts about this diet is that it includes easy to find everyday products that you don't have to spend a fortune on or look high and low to find. More than likely, you'll have all of these in your cupboard anyway. It's more a process of eliminating other foods and products, than it is about trying to find these new ones. This makes it a diet that is a lot easier to follow and more manageable to maintain.

You'll look great, and you'll be inspired to take on a healthy lifestyle. I cannot wait to hear how your journey has gone. Remember to be kind to yourself and to allow your body time to adjust to all the changes.

Lastly, be proud of this amazing first step you have taken!

Finally, if you enjoyed this book, then I'd like to ask you for a favor, would you be kind enough to leave a review for this book on Amazon? It'd be greatly appreciated!

Be sure to check out our website at www.thetotalevolution.com for more information.

Thank you!

OUR OTHER BOOKS

Below you'll find some of our other books that are popular on Amazon.com and the international sites.

The Dukan Diet: A High Protein Diet Plan To Lose Weight And Keep It Off For Life

Mayo Clinic Diet: A Proven Diet Plan For Lifelong Weight Loss

Glycemic Index Diet: A Proven Diet Plan For Weight Loss and Healthy Eating With No Calorie Counting

Clean Eating Diet: A 10 Day Diet Plan To Eat Clean, Lose Weight And Supercharge Your Body

Wheat Belly: The Anti-Diet - A Guide To Gluten Free Eating And A Slimmer Belly

IIFYM: Flexible Dieting - Sculpt The Perfect Body While Eating The Foods You Love

Mediterranean Diet: 101 Ultimate Mediterranean Diet Recipes To Fast Track Your Weight Loss & Help Prevent Disease

Acid Reflux Diet: A Beginner's Guide To Natural Cures And Recipes For Acid Reflux, GERD And Heartburn

Hypothyroidism Diet: Natural Remedies & Foods To Boost Your Energy & Jump Start Your Weight Loss

It Starts With Food: A 30 Day Diet Plan To Reset Your Body, Lose Weight And Become A Healthier You

Made in the USA
Thornton, CO
09/21/22 15:06:34

f56c034f-c538-4c05-a862-a85a7bb68957R01